WHAT PEOPLE ARE SAYING ABOUT

There Is Life After Breast Cancer

Courageous, bold, powerful, authentic, godly woman of strength and perseverance—Rena Tarbet resonates an awe-inspiring, real-life picture of what genuine character under crisis looks like. Her response to the thief named cancer did not rob her of hope or faith, but rather built an increased mountain of both. It did not rob her of a wildly successful career or ever-growing quality family time. It didn't rob her of joy or dignity. It's true that you don't know how strong you are until you have to find out; and it's true that you're not fully tested until disease beyond your control or understanding inhabits your own physical body. I've never known anyone to so fiercely face cancer or other crisis, sold out and determined to beat it! Determined to win with gratitude and purpose! If you or a loved one just got hit with a surprise diagnosis, and you're wondering if you can get through it, this is a must-read! Rena will have you laughing and crying but optimistic and hope-filled about your own expanded purpose. Her shared experiences will ignite a determination inside of you to *live* abundantly through the journey to an even more meaningful season ahead. She has paved the way as *none* other, and her story, tenacity, faith, genuine love, and concern for you will stop you in your tracks and cause you to find your own voice more powerfully. You're not alone. Rena has been there, and been there again. I'm confident this book will make a difference in how you view what is ahead, and I know the way you view it in large part dictates the outcome. God bless you as He has blessed and used my friend Rena Tarbet to touch countless lives for the better.

Pamela Waldrop Shaw
Motivational Speaker
Independent National Sales Director, MKI

For well over thirty years I've heard my father, motivational icon Zig Ziglar, sing the praises of Rena Tarbet. He has called her exceptional, successful, a strong leader and an inspiration to all who know her. Because of his admiration and respect for her, I count the opportunity to read and endorse Rena's book *There is Life After Breast Cancer* a blessing. Her words of wisdom gleaned from years of personal experience with cancer are both comforting and a rallying cry to gear up for a victorious battle. Women who take her message to heart will have a huge head start on winning the fight for their life.

Julie Ziglar Norman
Founder of Ziglar Women, Author, Inspirational Speaker

I have had the privilege of hearing Rena Tarbet speak in front of thousands as she shares her tremendous story of success in the business world. Rena has a great way of reaching her audience, weaving hysterical stories with insightful wisdom. Her messages are delivered with courage, honesty, and an uplifting spirit in a way unique to Rena. Everyone will benefit from reading her words as they are about life's challenges, moving forward in spite of them, and her endurance. Rena's positive attitude, gratefulness, and faith amidst the most daunting circumstances, new diagnoses, and years of setbacks come through on each page. You'll especially enjoy the reflections she writes at the end of each Chapter—they are devotionals revealing an unshakable faith. I've benefited greatly from this book and I know that you'll be blessed by it as well.

Bob Stoops
Head Coach/University of Oklahoma Football Team

Like many others, my family has been impacted by this awful disease. I just wish that my mother had been able to read a book like this as she fought her battle with breast cancer.

Jim Underwood, MA, MBA, DBA
Bestselling author of The Ethics Trap *and* More Than a Pink Cadillac

I have had the honor of caring for Rena Tarbet as her physician assistant and being able to call her my friend for most of her cancer journey. I thought I knew everything about her, but after reading *There is Life After Breast Cancer*, I find a poignant story of her heartfelt emotions both in fighting the disease and embracing the life she so loves. She is an inspiration to all who know her, and I believe everyone who reads *There is Life After Breast Cancer* will also find the inspiration necessary to embark on the journey of breast cancer. This is a must-read for every woman diagnosed with breast cancer and for their families and friends. It is written by a woman who truly talks the talk and walks the walk.

Mary Kippa,
PA-C

On rare occasions in life, you may cross paths with an individual who epitomizes the inner strength of steel in the face of extreme adversity. Rena is one such individual. As if a diagnosis of cancer is not enough, challenges of mitigating the untoward consequences of treatment in the early days of her journey were daunting. Rena faced and still faces with rare courage what has been meted out to her. It was not uncommon for Rena to finish a treatment of chemotherapy and fly to a distant city to deliver a motivational speech, knowing that the travel would be a physical challenge. I vividly remember asking her, "Rena, why don't you take a day off since you just finished chemotherapy?" And her determined response would be, "I can throw up just as well on the airplane as I can at home." This one statement speaks volumes of her courage and determination to fight the battle of cancer and prevail over the enemy while still living her life. This very candid outpouring of her sentiments in *There is Life After Breast Cancer* is a rare opportunity for the reader. In addition to a chronology of her courageous battle, this book will be motivation for all.

Dr. Amanullah Khan, M.D., Ph.D.

There Is *life* After Breast Cancer

OTHER BOOKS AVAILABLE FROM PLAN B BOOKS

The Significance Breakthrough: The One Thing that Can Change Your Work, Your Relationships, and Your Life

Character and Success: 6 Traits That Will Transform Your Relationships

The Ethics Trap: How "Situational Ethics" Can Destroy Your Life and Your Business

The Challenge: How Pride and Self-Deceit Destroy Our Hope, Joy, and Success

YourVirtualBookstore.com

There Is *life* After Breast Cancer

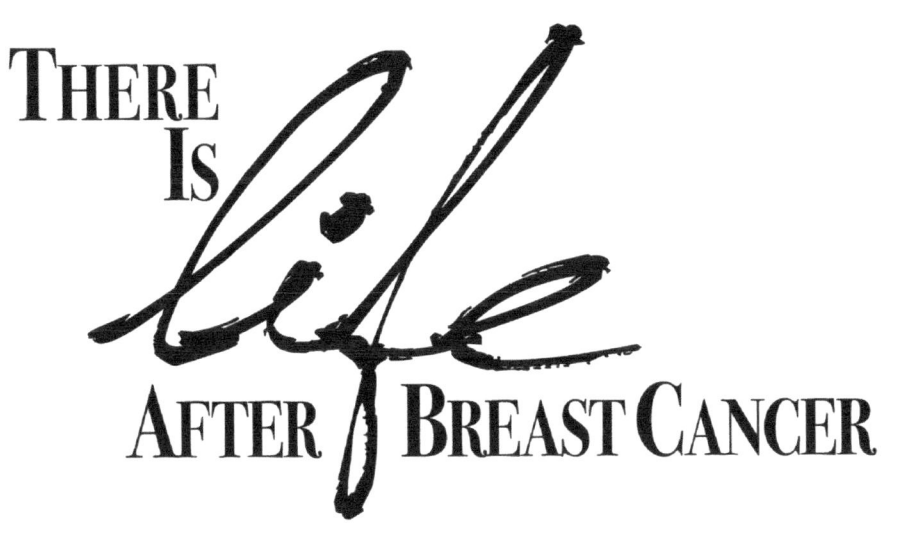

HOW TO RECLAIM YOUR LIFE AND LIVE IT ABUNDANTLY

RENA TARBET

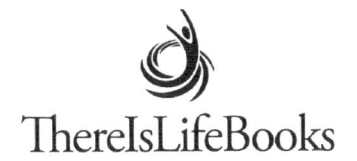

ThereIsLifeBooks

A Division of Plan B Book Publishing
Southlake, TX 76092
YourVirtualBookstore.com

There Is Life after Breast Cancer
Copyright © 2012 Rena Tarbet

All rights reserved. This book may not be duplicated or reproduced in any form or manner whatsoever, except as allowed by the U.S. Copyright Act of 1976, as amended, without the prior and express written permission of the publisher.

Published by

> There Is Life Books
> A Division of Plan B Book Publishing
> 2707 N. Carroll Avenue
> Southlake, TX 76092

Visit our website: YourVirtualBookstore.com

Unless otherwise noted, Scripture quotations are from the New King James Version (NKJV), copyright ©1979, 1980, 1982, Thomas Nelson, Inc., Publishers. Used by permission.

Ten percent of all book sales will be donated to the Mary Kay Foundation and its efforts to eliminate cancers affecting women.

ISBN: 978-0-9837861-9-1

Printed in the United States of America
11 12 13 14 15 16 TDP 6 5 4 3 2 1

Contents

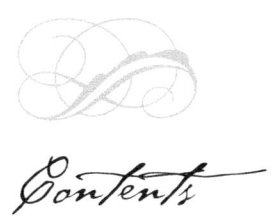

Introduction vii

1 Life Is Full of Surprises 1

2 Coping with Grief 9

3 Accepting Life's Challenges 17

4 Bouncing Back 25

5 The Value of Endurance 33

Epilogue: Just One More Thing 43

Recommended Reading 45

About the Author 47

Introduction

A most unwelcome aspect of dealing with a serious illness is that it almost always interferes with our plans and changes the direction of our lives in ways we could never have anticipated. In 1975, before I detected a small lump in my breast, I was in a good place. I was happy and productive, with a loving husband and three great kids. My business was thriving, and I was on my way to bigger and better things.

I had grown up in a happy home in south Texas, not far from San Antonio. My parents didn't have a lot of money, but what we lacked in material comforts we made up for with strong family values and hardheaded determination. I always believed that good things happen to good people, and there were many good things in my life.

I'd had a successful high school career. I was popular, made good grades, participated in varsity tennis and other sports, and I received all kinds of recognition for my activities. I was elected president of my the FHA, FTA, and captain of the drill team, and I was dating the young man who would soon be my husband.

INTRODUCTION

Eddie Tarbet and I were married shortly after I graduated from high school, and I began my lifelong dream of being a devoted homemaker and a good Christian wife.

While Eddie was in college, completing a master's degree in social work, I did my best to stretch our meager income of just three hundred dollars a month, trying to make ends meet. I was pretty good at that, but I couldn't help wondering what else I might be missing. I liked having lots of friends around, a busy schedule of activities, and I especially liked being recognized as a leader.

Making the transition from high school to married life was going to be a bigger adjustment than I had anticipated. Keeping up with our children, Jeff, Kim, and Brian, could be challenging. They were normal, healthy kids who were full of energy and into everything kids like to do. But I was ready for a new challenge, and that's when a dear friend who was a beauty consultant opened a door for me to a whole new world!

I took a few baby steps into that world in the beginning. But suddenly I was seeing new things, new people, new ideas, and I realized this was something I wanted to do. Before long I was off and running, and by age thirty-two, I was flying. I had a career that gave me tremendous pleasure and satisfaction. Our income had increased substantially, we had moved to a new home, and I was happier than I had ever been.

Then one evening, just as I was getting ready for bed, I felt the lump under my arm. There are few things in life as frightening as a diagnosis of cancer. Cancer is an enemy that strikes when you least

Introduction

expect it and changes your life in the most unpredictable and inconvenient ways. Eddie and I weren't terribly worried about the lump in my breast at first. We were told that 95 percent of lumps are benign, and many don't require surgery of any kind. However, to be cautious, I checked with our family doctor and followed his advice to have the lump examined by a surgeon.

After a mammogram and needle biopsy, both of which were negative, the surgeon advised me to have the lump removed, just to be safe. But when I woke up from the operation, I discovered that the medical team had been surprised to find that the lump was, in fact, malignant, and in danger of spreading. While I was still under sedation, my husband gave consent for the surgery, and the doctor went ahead and performed a modified radical mastectomy of my left breast.

Making the Adjustment

It's difficult to describe the combination of shock, fear, and indignation I felt when they told me what had just happened. The surgeon was at my bedside along with Eddie and one of my closest friends, all of them with tears in their eyes. None of us had seen this coming, but when I had time to think about it, I realized that the doctors had only taken that step because they believed it was essential to save my life. Now, thirty-six years later, I know they made the right decision.

Unfortunately, breast cancer is the most common cancer among women in the United States. It is also one of the leading causes of cancer death among women. According to the most recent statistics from the Centers for Disease Control and Prevention (CDC), more than 200,000

Introduction

American women are diagnosed with breast cancer each year. Approximately 20 percent of those women will lose their battle with cancer, which is tragic. But the good news is that the remaining 80 percent are able to survive, to fight the disease successfully, often for years, and a remarkable number of cases are able to go into complete remission.

Thanks to new scientific discoveries and improved understanding of these types of cancer, the number of new cases of breast cancer has been in decline for the past dozen years or so. The number of new cases dropped by 2 percent between 1998 and 2007—that's more than four thousand fewer cases. That may seem like a small improvement, but it is a positive step forward, and the numbers will likely fall even further as researchers continue to explore new and better options for prevention and treatment.

Meanwhile, there are many things that women diagnosed with breast cancer can do to improve the prognosis. An eleven-year study of 2,200 women diagnosed with breast cancer by medical researchers at the University of California, San Francisco, found that those who continued doing normal, everyday activities after breast cancer treatment did much better and lived longer than those who did not.

In addition, the CDC reports that women with strong social ties—especially to their husbands, children, and other family members—do much better than women with weak ties with family and friends. Dr. Meira Epplein of Vanderbilt University reported that women who score high in social well-being show a 38 percent reduction in the risk of death. They also show a 48 percent reduction in the risk for breast cancer's return.

Introduction

That's the kind of news I really appreciate, because I've never been the kind of person to take bad news lying down. Over the past thirty-five years, I have mounted a campaign against this disease, using every weapon I can find to defeat it. With the loving support of my husband and family, the skillful and dedicated treatment provided by my doctors, and the unfailing care and attention of so many friends who make up my extended family, I'm still going, and more determined than ever to prove that there is hope. There is life after breast cancer, and that's the reason I have written this book.

In the following pages I want to offer hope and encouragement for all those who have been touched by this disease. I will not pretend that the journey through this valley is going to be easy, because it isn't. There are risks on every side, and I have no desire to trivialize them. However, you don't have to be a victim. There will be days when you feel like giving up—sometimes the medical treatments can make you feel that way—but you can push through those feelings to the other side. You can decide whether you will allow yourself to be defeated by the disease or will accept the challenge to fight back and live a full and productive life, despite the illness.

There's hope because of the medical and scientific breakthroughs that are just around the corner. I'm convinced we are going to defeat this disease, once and for all, very soon. The science is on our side. But there's also hope because a big part of this journey is psychological and emotional. In other words, you can improve your situation and your chances of recovery if you refuse to be defeated by your doubts.

Those who lose hope, who let themselves believe it's futile to keep

Introduction

on fighting, or who react to the expressions of concern of their friends and family with self-pity and sorrow will be at a big disadvantage. A certain amount of grief and sadness is inevitable: I don't want to pretend you won't experience those feelings from time to time. But those who accept the challenge, knowing it's going to be a struggle, will find within themselves all the resources they need to conquer their fears and live every minute with enthusiasm and hope.

I do want to say one little thing about the arrangement of this book. At the end of each section, you will find a special note from me to you that I call "Reflections." Because I've been there, I know how discouraged we can become in fighting this dreadful disease. With that in mind, I wanted you to have a personal message at the end of each section that is meant just for you. I hope and pray that you will find them encouraging and uplifting.

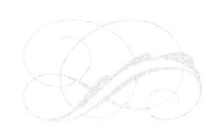

Reflections

My dear friend,

I hope that I can be of some help, strength, and encouragement because I have also battled this disease for more than thirty years. During these years, my treatments included radiation, cobalt, surgeries, and several consecutive years of chemo. I just want you to know that your story can be a victorious one too.

I'll be the first to admit that I don't have all the answers. I've run into my share of obstacles over the years, but I believe what the Bible says: "All things work together for good to those who love God, to those who are the called according to His purpose" (Romans 8:28). Just know that God has a purpose for each of us, in sickness and in health, and He will see us through. Together we must learn to do everything in our power to overcome our trials and disappointments, and then leave the rest to Him.

I love the Bible verse that says, "We are more than conquerors through Him who loved us" (Romans 8:37). That is such a wonderful promise. With faith, all things are possible, and regardless what kinds of challenges life may throw at us, we have the assurance that God's love is real. He is with us through the darkest night, and He has already given us the power to rise above our circumstances and overcome our limitations.

Reflections

It is my sincerest wish for you to take that promise as a challenge and, by the choices you make from here on, prove that your life is worth living, even after a diagnosis of breast cancer!

Love and Belief,

Rena

1
Life Is Full of Surprises

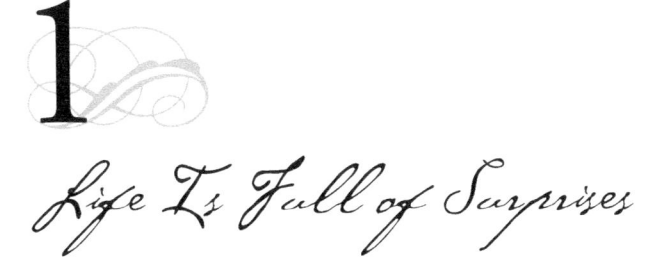

We will probably never know in this life why accidents happen or why some people suffer while others seem to sail through life in relative ease and comfort. Unfortunately, life doesn't come with a guarantee. It would be nice if we could simply take out an insurance policy to make sure we never have to experience pain or sorrow. But it doesn't work that way. For most of us, life is a mixture of good and bad news, and there are times when the only news we hear is bad. We don't get to make the rules, but we don't have to accept everything that life throws at us either.

For many people, the first response to a cancer diagnosis is disbelief. We refuse to accept it. We think cancer is something that only happens to other people. But that can be a dangerous mistake. It is very important to take news like that seriously, especially when it's bad news, and one of the first things we need to do is to begin looking for constructive ways to deal with the situation. Delaying the response, in most cases, will only make matters worse, and denial can be fatal. So once you have a good idea what you're up against, you need to take steps to deal with it.

I never want to be controlled by my circumstances. I made up my mind a long time ago to stand up to my problems and, to the best of my ability, to take ownership of my own situation. I've said it this way in the past: "The quality of our lives depends not on what happens *to* us but what happens *in* us." We can adapt to bad news and transform it in positive ways, if we respond appropriately. We all have the power to transform a negative situation into a positive learning experience, if we're willing to stand our ground.

One of the first things I did after my surgery was to start asking questions. I wanted to know what the surgeons knew about my condition, and I wanted to know the prognosis. At that point, I wanted to learn everything I could about this disease that would help me get back on my feet and make a speedy recovery. I had always believed that good things happen to good people, but I learned that bad things can happen to good people, too, and life-threatening illnesses can happen even in the best of families.

Life isn't always fair, but that doesn't mean we have to accept defeat gracefully. So during my hospital stay, I decided I wanted to take charge of my life and get back to work. I love doing business, and I love talking with people about the beauty products and services we offer. I had friends and clients all over the country, so I asked an assistant to bring my Rolodex and my appointment book to my room, and I set up an office right there in my hospital bed.

At first, my doctors thought I was hopped-up on speed, because I

Life Is Full of Surprises

was going on with my life as if nothing had happened. Some people probably thought I'd gone over the edge. When my best friend saw those things beside my bed, she had them removed while I was sleeping. But I got them back as soon as I awoke, and I told everybody I had work to do. I knew that I wasn't going to get better if I simply lay there in that hospital room feeling sorry for myself. The doctors assured me they had gotten rid of the cancerous cells, so my job now was to let the healing begin and get back to normal as soon as possible. For me, normal was a busy workday, speaking to my friends, family, and clients on the telephone.

I knew what I needed to do. I needed to start thinking creatively about how I would proceed from that moment on and how I would go about pursuing my daily goals. I wasn't about to let negative thoughts and self-pity take control of my life. I was successful in business because I was a highly motivated person, and I was a motivator for hundreds of other women. It's much easier to keep a positive mental attitude when we have something good to look forward to, and there were so many good things in my life.

THE LONG CAMPAIGN

Over the next few years, I not only continued to grow in my career, but I became a sort of medical encyclopedia. I made it a point to learn everything I could about the medical, nutritional, mental, and spiritual aspects of the situation in which I found myself. By 1979, I still had a positive attitude, and I had begun looking into the possibility of reconstructive surgery.

But nothing I learned lessened the blow of a second diagnosis, when I discovered that the cancer was back and had spread to my right breast. Suddenly, everything I had assumed was up for grabs. I struggled with the news for a while, but once the shock had worn off, my reflexes kicked in, and I was ready for battle. After a simple mastectomy of my right breast, I was still optimistic. I felt we were winning the battle and I had finally beaten the odds.

Before long my attitude rebounded, and my life was returning to normal when, one year later, I found out the cancer had spread to my bones. Up to that point I had resisted most of the radical treatments the doctors had recommended. I knew enough about chemotherapy to know I didn't want to go there if I didn't have to; but with this new diagnosis, I understood that the time had finally come.

The side effects of chemotherapy are notoriously bad. That much I knew, and the thought of losing my hair and dealing with nausea and other issues was frightening. But, once again, I decided to prepare myself by learning everything I could about the various treatment facilities in the Southwest. If I was going to submit to this new indignity, then I wanted to find the place with the best reputation and the best record of success. I was determined I was going to beat this disease once and for all!

It's easy to lose hope when you're in the middle of a long, hard struggle with cancer. Doing my research and deciding on the best treatment center was my way of maintaining control. Sometimes people with serious illnesses come to the conclusion that things are so out of control they have no choice. After doing everything they know

Life Is Full of Surprises

how to do, preparing mentally and praying for recovery, the disease just keeps coming back, and they succumb to depression, fear, and guilt. At that point, they give up and allow their doctors, family, or someone else to make all the decisions regarding the types of therapy they will undergo. They simply do as they're told, as if they have no say in what's happening.

That's not an uncommon reaction, but it does not have to be the case. Even in the most difficult situations, there are always options, and the patient needs to be involved in these vital decisions. In my case, I decided to fly down to the M.D. Anderson Cancer Research Center in Houston, Texas, to begin chemotherapy treatments. Those treatments have continued in one form or another for years now. But thanks to a suggestion from a good friend—along with the advice of a wise and compassionate physician I encountered quite by chance while visiting my friend and mentor, Mary Kay Ash, at a hospital in Dallas—I added a variety of new treatment options to my routine.

I haven't stopped fighting the disease, and I don't plan to stop, even when I'm declared sound and in complete remission. In fact, I'm more committed to the challenge today than ever before. What I've learned with the help of my physician is that successful treatment of cancer involves multiple disciplines. There is no one-size-fits-all treatment. All patients need personalized treatment routines tailored to their individual needs and desires.

In some cases, that may mean a combination of radiation therapy and chemotherapy, along with changes in diet and exercise routines. One of the most promising diagnostic tools today is the positron emission tomography (PET) scan, used to examine all the vital organs of the body. This imaging technology is helpful in locating and diagnosing cancers. The PET scan can actually tell the difference between benign and malignant cells, and it can detect whether or not the disease has moved from one part of the body to another. The point is, every option should be on the table, and I didn't rule out anything.

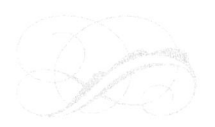

Reflections

My dear friend,

I think I have a good idea what you might be experiencing right now, because the one thing that almost suffocated me after my initial diagnosis was the feeling of hopelessness. Is that what you're feeling? Before you read another word, I want you to know, right now in this very moment, that there is hope! I so wish I could sit down and talk with you, because I want you to know that I do understand the uncertainty and fear that you may be feeling.

Would it surprise you to know that many people have been victorious in their own battles against cancer simply because they had seen others win the battle too? That was an important shift in my thinking and made a huge difference in how I fought the disease. This is the time you need to anchor your mind to the truth. *If* they *can win,* you *can win too!*

I pray that you will find your own hope stirred as you read my letters to you. These Reflections are my own thoughts put to paper of my march through the various steps of fear, depression, recovery, and then hope. Just as I did, you will soon realize that your feeling of despair is simply a steppingstone to a great and

Reflections

wonderful hope that will carry you through your journey. You will also become aware that only you can own this journey, because very few people may understand what you're going through or how you feel. Likewise, you own the victory, my friend!

Faithfully Yours,

Rena

2

Coping with Grief

As a business owner, beauty consultant, and motivational speaker, I've had the privilege of speaking to thousands of women over the last thirty-five years about fulfilling their dreams. Many of those women listened to what I had to say and went on to successful careers of their own. During those presentations, I frequently shared with the audience a lesson I had learned from Mary Kay Ash many years before, which was, "Beauty is both what's on the inside, as well as what's on the outside." That's an important lesson, and I believe it with all my heart. But my battle with cancer had turned into all-out war. I was a fighter, but there were many days when I felt I was anything but beautiful.

Losing my hair was one of the most depressing experiences of my life. I think that must be true for any woman in that situation. The doctors had told me what would happen, but that didn't make it any easier. Every morning when I woke up, I would find clumps of hair on my pillow. I couldn't run a comb or brush through my hair without taking out even more. I prepared for the inevitable by buying several attractive wigs. Then one evening, before I was scheduled to leave for a very special trip to Spain, my family and I gathered around the dining table to pluck out the last strands of my hair.

It was an emotional moment for all of us, and I'll never forget my daughter, Kim, running into the kitchen to get a baggie in which to put the hair. As she was stuffing clumps into that little plastic sack, she looked at me with tears in her eyes and said, "Mommy, I love you anyway!" Those were very special words, and they've been a constant reminder that my family's love for me is unchanging, hair or no hair. Regardless what physical or emotional hurdles I may have to jump over in my battle with cancer, my family is always there for me, and they love me unconditionally!

The greatest surprise of that episode, however, was that I wasn't just losing the hair on my head. I was losing every hair on my body, including my eyebrows and eyelashes, which was another shock. I did my best to deal with every surprise, but I have to admit that it was one of the lowest points in my struggle with cancer, and at various times I found myself on the edge of full-blown depression.

I refused to give in to the temptation to feel sorry for myself; it was a struggle, but I knew that was a dead-end street. Then at one point, I read an article about the predictable cycle of grief that often comes with this sort of illness. A Swiss-American psychiatrist named Elisabeth Kübler-Ross wrote a book entitled *On Death and Dying* that describes the five stages of grief. The stages include denial, anger, bargaining, depression, and acceptance. Not everyone goes through all of them, she said, and people don't necessarily experience these emotions in the same way. But I thought her findings were insightful, and I would like to describe the five stages here, to help those struggling with this illness to identify some of the emotions they may be feeling.

Stage 1: Denial

For many people, their first reaction to a diagnosis of cancer is disbelief and denial. They want to believe it's not true, that somebody has made a big mistake. Actually, this is a good thing, because denial is a way of coping with the stress of a negative diagnosis. We tend to think that denial is merely refusing to accept reality, but researchers have found that it is nature's way of protecting us from despair. Denial helps us pace our feelings until the reality of our situation settles in. But it's only the first stage. Before long the feelings and fears we've been suppressing begin to emerge, and that leads to the second stage.

Stage 2: Anger

Dr. Kübler-Ross found that, much to her surprise, anger is an essential stage of the healing process. Most people tend to think that anger is inappropriate, an over-reaction, or some form of selfishness, but in this case anger is actually a sign of strength. It means you want and expect answers, and your mind begins focusing anger on every possible target for the crisis you're facing, from God to your family, your doctors, yourself, and even life itself. Anger at the weakness you're dealing with is a sign of an intense desire to live. You want to be free, to move on with your life, and that's a very important step in recovering from any kind of loss. At that point, you begin moving toward the next stage.

STAGE 3: BARGAINING

In the early stages of an illness, your mind is racing, looking for a way out. The first step for many people involves bargaining with God for a reprieve. Some will say, "God, if you take this disease away, I'll never say or do anything bad ever again!" There are, of course, many verses to that song. But if the condition persists, the individual enters the "What if?" cycle, followed by the "If only . . . " cycle. We're looking for answers, and we may try to make a deal with our illness or with the pain we're feeling. But when that doesn't work, we collapse slowly and surely into the next stage.

STAGE 4: DEPRESSION

For whatever reasons, none of the prayers, strategies, or mind tricks we've tried have given us the relief we so earnestly desire. Even though prayer has helped in some ways, giving us a sense of God's presence, and while the treatments we've received may be making the pain bearable and the progress of the illness less severe, we're beginning to lose hope, wondering if things will ever get better. Even if the physical pain is under control, the emotional pain is getting worse. At some point, we begin to think *Why fight it? Who am I kidding? I may as well give up.*

Friends and family say they're there for us, of course, and they offer encouragement, but for a long time we simply can't accept those promises, and depression sets in. Eventually, however, we move through this "dark night of the soul" toward acceptance and a renewed sense of determination to fight back and take charge of our situations. The timeframe varies, of course, from one individual to the next, but relief will eventually come. For those with a strong Christian faith, the process can happen very quickly. Our hope is restored. But it is important to understand that occasional lapses into depression are not a sign of weakness; they are part of a natural healing process and a way of moving past the grief.

Stage 5: Acceptance

Acceptance should not be confused with giving up and accepting defeat. It is not surrender, and it is not a weakening of the will to fight. Rather, it is a sign that we have come to grips with the diagnosis, and we've gained a better understanding of the battle that lies ahead. We've looked at the situation from all angles and found what some have described as "the new normal." Once we reach that point, we're ready to move on, to listen to the advice of doctors, nutritionists, therapists, and others, and make our own decisions.

For some people, acceptance may simply mean having more good days than bad ones. But instead of denying our feelings, we're now willing to listen to others, to think about tomorrow and the next day after that, to put most of our fears behind us and move on. Friendship suddenly matters more than ever, and we feel a renewed and deepening love for the spouse, children, loved ones, and colleagues who have stood by us all along. Even in the midst of our struggles, we can be reasonably content, knowing that whatever else may happen, we're in it to win it.

There Is Life After Breast Cancer

What I've learned through my own battle with cancer is that it's always best to be pro-active, to listen to those who have wisdom to share, and to approach each new challenge in the belief that things will get better soon. And when I'm at my weakest, I've learned to rely on my family and friends for support.

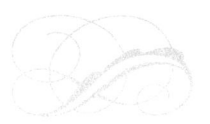

Reflections

My dear friend,

I want you to know that I do understand what you are going through right now. I will never forget my early days of dealing with cancer. I had thought that the battle would be with the disease and the pain associated with my treatments. Little did I know that the real battle would be with my fear, discouragement, and depression.

This is the very reason I want to come along side you and to be the friend who has already traveled this path. It is my sincerest wish to be a companion as well as a mentor to you. By the same token, I want to pass along to you something that I learned from my mentor, Mary Kay Ash. She never let me give up. She never allowed me to consider failure. She was always there for me and for everyone else in our organization calling out, "Keep on keeping on!"

I want to be completely honest with you that my journey wasn't always a mountaintop experience. Yes, there were times that I "hit bottom." My suspicion is that you'll hit bottom too. It's one thing to put up a good front when family and friends are there, but it's an entirely different thing when you wake up alone at midnight in a hospital bed, and all you can think about is a

Reflections

frightful and unsure future. Take a moment to think on these words:

"Hear me, Lord, and have mercy on me. Help me, O Lord. You have turned my mourning into joyful dancing. You have taken away my clothes of mourning and clothed me with joy that I might sing praises to you and not be silent. O Lord my God, I will give you thanks forever!" (Psalm 30:10-12)

I so hope you will take the time when you get to that point to spend a few moments with the Lord. My prayer for you is that He will give you a heart to "keep on keeping on."

Faithfully yours,

Rena

# 3
Accepting Life's Challenges

Once I understood what my challenges were going to be, I made a conscious decision to wage an all-out war on the disease that had invaded my life so abruptly. I wanted to be strong, so I laid out my plans as a general prepares for combat. But like it or not, even on my best days there were times when I was nearly paralyzed with fear. Sometimes we react to bad news with fear simply because we don't know enough; at other times we're afraid because of something we've overheard. And sometimes we're afraid because the challenge is just so enormous. At times I wrestled with all of these.

There were times in the early stages of my illness when friends or acquaintances would say something that hurt me deeply. They weren't trying to hurt me, of course; in fact, they were trying to cheer me up, but their words had the opposite effect than what they intended. Each time something like that happened, I had to remind myself that I was in charge of my attitudes. I was not a victim. I was determined to beat that illness, and I wasn't about to let fear, misunderstanding, or resentment take control of my life.

Fear is a powerful emotion that operates independently of our conscious minds. Most of the time we have little control over our fears, because, like denial, fear is nature's way of protecting us from harm. Fear can be helpful in some situations: we ought to be afraid of fire, sharp objects, angry people, automobile accidents, and things of that sort. That's healthy fear. But fear can also be false and unfounded, and if our fear comes simply because of ignorance or lack of knowledge, it can slow down the healing process. Doctors tell us that irrational fear can lead to increased stress and anxiety, which not only hamper the healing process, but can also contribute to other conditions and increase the medical risks.

One acronym of fear is "false evidence appearing real." We let a little bit of information lead us to false conclusions, and we lose confidence in our ability to resist. When faced with a sudden bout of fear, we have two options: we can either give in to the fear and withdraw into ourselves, or we can refuse to be intimidated and fight to get back in control of the situation. I occasionally use the expression, "Fake it till you make it." Sometimes you have to put up a good front to convince yourself that you're not afraid; and if you do that, before long you'll probably discover that you're really not afraid anymore.

My greatest fear during the early days of my illness was the fear of the unknown. There are no two people with precisely the same condition or symptoms. There are no two people with precisely the same treatment options. What if the doctors misdiagnosed my illness? What if they were giving me bad advice? As I was learning about my condition, I imagined all sorts of things that could go wrong, things

Accepting Life's Challenges

that could rob me of my security, or take away all the wonderful things I enjoyed so much. Those were painful times, but I eventually found ways to overcome those feelings and take charge of my emotions.

Sometimes I would pull out my notepad and write down my thoughts, questions, and fears. When I put them down in black and white, I was able to focus on my concerns much more easily and respond to them in a logical way. Those notebooks became part of my prayer time, as I read each line and prayed about it, sharing my fears and concerns with God. It was miraculous how He took my worries away, one by one, and gave me a new sense of peace. In many cases, my fears melted away; but in those that were more complicated, I could ask the medical staff for answers. And in every case I had the knowledge that, whatever happened, my life was in God's hands, and He was there with me in my distress.

Keeping On Keeping On

One of the most important elements in any kind of therapy is time. If you accidentally cut your finger, it may hurt for a minute or two, but it will heal in time. The human body is made that way, and there are many things in life that can only get better with time. Unfortunately, that's not a popular message in this age of iPhones, GPS devices, and microwave ovens. We want everything to be fast and easy, but that's rarely possible with serious medical problems. Now and then God may choose to heal an individual suddenly and miraculously; we all hope and pray for that. But even when He doesn't heal us that way, our bodies are working around the clock to restore us to good health, and that's a miracle too.

The ancient Greek physician, Hippocrates—often called the "father of medicine"—stressed that "healing takes time." It doesn't matter whether it's a physical illness or a complicated emotional issue, recovery of any kind takes time, and while time is working its magic in combination with the magical healing properties of the human body, it's important to remain positive and hopeful, awaiting the outcome. Or as I often say, you've got to keep on keeping on.

In 1 Corinthians 13:13, the final verse of the great "love chapter" in the New Testament, the apostle Paul wrote, "Now abide faith, hope, and love; these three, but the greatest of these is love." Those words are among the most essential building blocks of the Christian life. Faith begins with the knowledge that God loves us and has a purpose for our life, and it includes the good news that Jesus came into the world and gave his life for our sins, not by accident, but because He loves us with an eternal love. We really need faith like that to carry on a long and demanding campaign against cancer, but we also need a strong sense of hope to give us the motivation to keep on fighting. Taken together, faith, hope, and love are powerful medicine.

Like time, hope is essential for healing to take place. Without hope we become victims of our doubts and fears, but when hope is strong in us, we have peace of mind and a sense of anticipation, believing that good things will happen. *Hope* means "living in the expectation of a favorable outcome," and the Bible tells us that God wants us to be *filled* with hope. As Paul wrote, "Now may the God of hope fill you with all joy and peace in believing, that ye may abound in hope, through the power of the Holy Spirit" (Romans 15:13). From begin-

Accepting Life's Challenges

ning to end, the Bible assures us that God is a God of hope, and He wants us to be completely filled with hope.

Accepting life's challenges means that you have looked at the options and decided to go forward in the hope of a positive outcome. There's not much anyone can do for someone who has lost hope. It's sad to see a man or woman who has given up and become dispirited by the effort of fighting their illness. Even though they believe in the power of prayer, they've lost hope. They succumb to doubts and fears and begin to believe they will never get better. Proverbs 13:12 says, "Hope deferred makes the heart sick." Losing hope only makes the situation worse.

It's so important to keep a positive attitude in your struggles, and every person doing battle with an illness of any kind must keep hope alive and vibrant. Most of us have heard the expression, "Where there's life there's hope." I believe that's true, but I also believe the reverse of that is true as well: "Where there's hope there's life!" Hope determines our actions, and actions determine the outcome. What better motivation can there be to keep hope alive?

Reflections

My dear friend,

At some point in the process of dealing with breast cancer, you may hit a "big wall." Sure, there are little walls along the way, too, but sooner or later you will find yourself facing a challenge that may seem even bigger than the fright and fear that rule the early days of dealing with the disease. The "big wall" is when you start coming to grips with the reality we all face as human beings: your own mortality.

As I think back through those days and how I dealt with the big wall, I must confess that I had the same fears and concerns that most everyone else has. One of the false ideas that people often have is that God will take away your fear. Perhaps that sounds really wonderful, but it would actually be completely disastrous in battling the disease. For example, a professional boxer creates strategies for defeating his opponent because he's conscious of what his opponent can do in the ring. Just like the boxer, we can use a healthy fear to focus our energy on a plan of action—a plan that does not ask God to remove the fear but asks Him to carry us through it.

I also want to talk to you about grieving. No one chooses sorrow, and no one should belittle you for a pe-

Reflections

riod of mourning. As I look back and think about how I went through the grieving process, it's clear to me that grieving is needed. Grieving is our way of coming to grips with and accepting the situation we are in. More than that, grieving takes us through the storm of uncertainty and into the warming rays of hope—a new confidence that is stronger and more powerful than we have ever experienced before.

After more than thirty years of victory over breast cancer, I remain resolute. There is life after breast cancer because there is hope! The challenges can change, and the treatments may vary, but we have hope. And because we have hope, we will be victorious!

Faithfully yours,

Rena

4
Bouncing Back

My battle with cancer was like a military campaign—a realistic description of what my family and I have been through. The first enemy attack came in 1974 without warning, but after the initial shock and surprise, we began mounting a fierce resistance. Then, with new and improved weapons and ammunition, we launched a relentless counterattack. Over the years, what I had hoped would be a brief skirmish and quick victory turned into a long and desperate siege. Many times I felt as if all hope was lost, but I fought on.

To begin with, I underwent two radical mastectomies four years apart, and a year later, I learned that the cancer had metastasized to my breastbone. Over the next two years, I underwent a grueling series of chemotherapy treatments. To make it easier to move around without being confined to my home or a hospital bed, I began wearing a small chemotherapy pump inside my clothing.

Later, I began a series of radiation treatments and a major change of diet with a nutritional program I discovered through the advice of a dear friend. But even with all those defensive measures, tests showed that the cancer had progressed from my sternum to my skull, and I underwent another round of radiation treatments to the area around my forehead. Finally, approximately four years later, I was officially declared to be in remission with no evidence of disease.

I had won another battle, and we celebrated, but we hadn't won the war. It was nearly ten years before the diagnosis changed once again. In a routine test, the doctors found new evidence of cancer in my skull, and they began increasing the chemotherapy dosages and trying new formulations that had only recently been approved by the Food & Drug Administration (FDA). Each time the oncologist prescribed a new treatment, we doubled up with a combination of chemotherapy and radiation treatments.

By 1999, twenty-five years after the battle had begun, a PET scan indicated that I was cancer free, with "no active disease." Accordingly, the chemotherapy treatments were scaled back, and I was given just one powerful drug at that time. But two years later, I began experiencing heart problems, possibly as a reaction to that drug. Then, in 2005, evidence revealed that new tumors were appearing.

Over the next ten years, I suffered further complications to my heart, liver, and brain. Off and on during all this time, I had been treated for bone lesions and a serious loss of bone density in my jaw. I even had a hysterectomy to prevent uterine cancer from developing. After so many vicious assaults, there were many times when my ability to fight back was severely limited. But I never gave up; I never gave in; I never quit fighting. The three things that have kept me on the frontlines of this military campaign have been my unflappable faith in a loving God, the encouragement of my loving family and supportive friends, and a large dose of hardheaded determination with which I was born.

Never, Never Give In

I'm sure you've heard the story, but it never fails to inspire me. In the fall of 1941, two months before the United States entered the Second World War, Nazi bombers were pulverizing English cities and towns. Many politicians and famous men were calling for England to surrender. The English prime minister, Winston Churchill, was a stubborn old warhorse known for his powerful speeches, which were often quite long, and he was calling for England to stand up courageously and continue the fight.

It was at this time that Sir Winston was asked to return to his old school to give a speech in honor of the young men who would be graduating that year. He was extremely busy as a leader of the British war effort, but he accepted the invitation, and everyone wondered what he would say. They expected a long, dry speech, explaining his position, but after a brief introduction, the old man stood up and spoke these words:

> This is the lesson: never give in, never give in, never, never, never, never—in nothing, great or small, large or petty—never give in except to convictions of honor and good sense. Never yield to force; never yield to the apparently overwhelming might of the enemy.

That was the entire speech, but he spoke with such intensity that many in the audience were shocked into silence. Then, when he sat back down, the hall erupted with applause. Everyone understood what he meant, and many historians say that speech—the shortest Sir Winston ever gave—probably changed the course of the war. Soon afterward, America joined the fight, and by 1945 Britain and her Allies were able to declare victory over the Nazis.

It wasn't the intensity of his words that made the speech so important, however, but the dignity, honor, and righteousness of the message. Now and then, a tyrant will come along and threaten us, using violence and insults and demanding surrender. But it's always wrong to give in to that kind of intimidation, and that's precisely how I've felt about the tyrant that invaded my body. I often feel that a whole squadron of Nazi bombers has hit me, but I'll never give up. I . . . will "never, never, never give in!"

From day one it has been one exhausting challenge after another, but I made a decision to resist with all the determination and resilience I could muster. Each new occurrence of the disease triggered powerful emotions, and there were days when all I could do was cry. But even during those days, what really hurt was seeing the sadness in the eyes of my loved ones. They hurt for me, but their love was strong, and they gave me renewed hope and strength.

I had invested all my energy in this struggle and, while I knew there was always the chance I might not come out of it alive, no one could say I didn't resist with every ounce of my strength. I've greeted each new diagnosis with a strategic response. To the chemotherapy and radiation treatments my doctors prescribed I added a new focus on diet and nutrition.

Following a suggestion from a good friend, I met with a nutritionist, who told me that changing my diet would contribute more to my eventual healing than any of those prescribed treatments, so I took his advice and eliminated pork, beef, sugar, salt, refined white flour, caffeine, and dairy products from my diet. That was another battle I had to fight for a while, but I added more fruits, vegetables, salads, and whole grains to my diet, along with lots of water, and I immediately began to feel better.

Along with those changes, I continued to focus on the mental and spiritual disciplines that had become so important to me. I devoured the Psalms and searched the Scriptures for words of hope and encouragement, and I felt God's presence. I call the individuals who gathered around me during this time my "Circle of Hope." My husband and children, my very special friends, my minister, and many of the teachers and leaders from our church, along with Dr. Amanullah Khan, who was my wise and faithful oncologist and hematologist, and the nurses who looked after me during my frequent hospital visits.

These were the people who were closest to me, and there were hundreds of friends and associates through my business who sent cards and notes or called or came by to see me. To be loved in that way is one of the most wonderful feelings in the world.

And I learned several important lessons from those experiences. One of the first was the importance of choosing your friends wisely. There are well-meaning people who will say nice things, but they always seem to be too busy when you need someone to talk to, or when you need a simple favor. I once heard someone say we will have many acquaintances but few real friends, and I believe that's true. We shouldn't expect everyone to care about our ups and downs, but we should treasure those who really care and who have a way of touching our hearts when we need it most. When my energy is low, those are the ones who always give me the strength to bounce back.

Reflections

My dear friend,

As I think about the battles I have fought over the years, two words keep coming to mind: perseverance and encouragement. As you know from reading this chapter, more than once or twice I've been faced with a cancer diagnosis. It's been one of the consistent occurrences in my life over the past thirty-plus years. One day it was breast cancer, then a few years later, it was cancer in my breastbone.

You know what? I'm still here! Every bleak or fearful circumstance I could think of in the end never materialized. Sure, I've continued to battle this illness, but you know what? I've been the winner in this battle for all these years! And I believe that inside of you is a winner too!

It is my hope that you will never view this as a time of disease or defeat. We are blessed with faithful friends, family, and caregivers, who will persevere and fight the battle with us. So when we think back on this journey, we'll remember the determination and encouragement of those who were by our side.

So hang tough, my friend. Do everything you know to do. Most importantly, fight with every fiber in your

Reflections

body and lean heavily upon God. He will always be with you in the battle.

Onward & Upward,

Rena

5
The Value of Endurance

In a long and frequently exhausting struggle for survival, nothing is more important than endurance. The writer of Hebrews says, "Let us lay aside every weight, and the sin which so easily ensnares us, and let us run with endurance the race that is set before us" (Hebrews 12:1). For me, the operative part of that verse is not just the idea of running a race but the importance of enduring hardship and eliminating every weight that can slow you down and keep you from reaching your goals. That verse means a lot to me because running with endurance has been my objective from the beginning.

When I first began this journey, I had to get past my natural defiance. I can be cantankerous at times, and I didn't want to accept a diagnosis of cancer. And then I didn't want to accept the prescriptions or the treatments the doctors were recommending. I thought that, somehow, through my own strength of will, I could beat the disease; after all, this wasn't supposed to happen to me. But that attitude didn't last very long, because cancer has a way of forcing us to pay attention and revert to a strong defensive position.

There Is Life After Breast Cancer

Once I accepted the fact that I had already had a radical mastectomy and that the risk of further complications was a distinct possibility, I realized I had to take an active role in the therapy I was given. As a motivational speaker and life-long high achiever, I decided to go after the disease with every weapon I could find. Medical treatments were fine, and I had plenty of those, but there were other resources I could draw upon as well. My faith was paramount: I couldn't have made it without the encouragement of the Scriptures. But I also began a persistent search for knowledge, reading countless books and articles, and talking to people who could shed new light on my condition.

My advice to anyone who is dealing with cancer is to use every option you can find to defeat this disease. Support groups help many people. There are groups for the families and friends of cancer patients, for their children, as well as for the patient. One of the best pieces of advice I ever received came from Dr. Khan, who advised me to live in the present. There's a tendency to fall back on the "what ifs" and "if onlys," thinking only about life before the disease began, or daydreaming about the future. But, as Dr. Khan assured me, taking it one day at a time is usually the best way to go.

In the darkest days of my struggle, I gained real strength from another practice that I strongly recommend: visualizing the healing process. I've described it as picturing the various medicines I was taking like little Pac-Man characters, racing through my cells, destroying all the cancerous tissue in my body. In the same way that an athlete can visualize a perfect golf swing or a perfect field goal, I could picture my body wiping out all those enemy cells and restoring my good health.

The Value of Endurance

Goal setting is another thing that has been tremendously important to me in my journey. In my motivational speeches, I often say, "If you don't know where you're going, how will you know when you get there?" That's what good, practical goal setting is all about. Make plans for the future, think about how you want to respond to your treatment, explore each of the options you're given, and decide how you want to proceed. Your doctors may have experience: they've seen how other patients respond, but you're unique. You need to decide what you want to accomplish, then make that your goal.

Lessons Learned

Cancer will challenge every fiber of your being, but you can overcome the challenges if you refuse to be defeated. In the computer world, I'm told, they use the expression, "Garbage in, garbage out," meaning that if you have bad information on the front end of a project you can't expect to produce good information at the conclusion. If you enter bad data, you'll get bad results. So good data is vitally important. During my illness, I learned a lot about myself, and I came to some conclusions I'd like to pass along to you.

Be pro-active in your own recovery. When you're dealing with a pernicious disease like cancer, you can't afford to let bad input spoil your chances for recovery, so you need to be pro-active in your search for good, practical information that will help you make a full recovery. Let your friends know that you're interested in learning more about treatment options and about new discoveries that may be helpful to you. Also, make sure your doctors understand that you're not sitting this one out on the sidelines: you want to be part of the team, and you want to be included in the decision-making process at each stage.

Don't dwell on the negative. Nothing is more defeating than a bad attitude. I've seen some people who are so overcome with grief after a disappointing diagnosis that they simply give up. Those folks don't last very long because they've decided their case is hopeless. But the fact is, you're never without hope. Even in the midst of your illness, there can be moments of joy. Even after a debilitating round of chemotherapy, you can find things to make you laugh. Even when you think you can't take another step, the friends and family walking beside you and holding you up can encourage you. Best of all, you can always rest in the assurance that, win or lose, God is there with you in the midst of your struggles.

Celebrate your victories. It's easy to develop a bad attitude when you're constantly being poked and prodded and examined as a laboratory specimen. It's easy to let anger and resentment rush over you like a tidal wave, but that's never a good idea. First of all, the men and women who are poking at you are only there because they have the skill to tackle this disease and improve your chances of recovery.

All along the way, you will have moments of victory, surprising achievements, and major improvements. Celebrate those victories, no matter how small. Radiate the happiness you feel to those around you. Laugh out loud. You'll be surprised how much better you'll feel with a little laughter. Just seeing you with such a positive attitude will make everyone in your circle want to work that much harder for your recovery.

The Value of Endurance

Prioritize the things you value. This is no surprise, but being diagnosed with breast cancer can change your whole worldview. Things that were very important to you before the diagnosis can fade into insignificance afterward. And things that meant little or nothing a few days or weeks ago suddenly become immensely important. Coming face to face with your own mortality will do that: but what better time to take a moment to think about the things that really matter to you and readjust your frame of reference. If you're like me, you'll probably decide that faith, family, and friends are at the top of your list while fame and fortune and all those creature comforts you once cared so much about are now much farther down the list. You'll have your own set of values to consider, but this will be an important step.

Make every minute count. When was the last time you told your spouse, children, parents, in-laws, or other special friends how much you love them? There are few things more important than that. Maybe you remember the scene in the movie, *The Wizard of Oz*, where Dorothy and her companions confronted the Wizard who had been hiding behind a screen. The Lion hoped the Wizard would give him courage, and the Scarecrow hoped to get a brain. But then, as the Wizard came out from behind the screen, he said to the Tin Man, "As for you, my galvanized friend, you want a heart. You don't know how lucky you are not to have one. Hearts will never be practical until they can be made unbreakable."

Somewhat surprised, the Tin Man replied, "But I still want one."

Before long, the Wizard took out a chain with a small heart dangling at the end. As he handed it to the Tin Man, he said, "So remember, my sentimental friend, a heart is not judged by how much you love, but by how much you are loved by others."

I've always liked that part of the story because it's a reminder that love is a two-way street. My mother used to say, "If you want friends, be friendly." What the Wizard was telling us is, if you want to be loved, let your loved ones know how much you care. I've never been a procrastinator, but I realized early in my illness that expressing my love for my family and friends was something I couldn't delay.

Do not grow weary. Of all the advice I've given in these pages, this may be the hardest to do. There are no easy days in the fight against breast cancer, and things that may have been simple for you at one time can suddenly seem next to impossible. Your energy is sapped, your will power is challenged, and your body is telling you to lie down and give up. Every one of these things can make you weary unless you daily lean on the Lord and pray for renewed strength. From day one, this has been my secret weapon.

In every situation, we can draw upon the Lord's strength. As the apostle Paul has written, in the final analysis, this is the true source of our hope. My prayer for each of you is that God will flood your heart with His love, renew your hope and strength, and guide you gently to a full and complete recovery. And I will leave you with these wonderful words from Paul:

> Therefore, since we have been made right in God's sight by faith, we have peace with God because of what Jesus Christ our Lord has done for us. Because of our faith, Christ has brought

The Value of Endurance

us into this place of undeserved privilege where we now stand, and we confidently and joyfully look forward to sharing God's glory.

We can rejoice, too, when we run into problems and trials, for we know that they help us develop endurance. And endurance develops strength of character, and character strengthens our confident hope of salvation. And this hope will not lead to disappointment. For we know how dearly God loves us, because he has given us the Holy Spirit to fill our hearts with his love. (Romans 5:1–5)

Reflections

My dear friend,

Today is the beginning of a new day and a new commitment to being the very best we can be. I realize that none of us know what tomorrow holds, but our comfort has to come from knowing who holds tomorrow! I just hope and pray that you'll place your faith in God, knowing Him as your personal savior and that you are clinging closely to that relationship during this difficult time. He alone can give you the strength, courage, and comfort that you need.

I have enjoyed more than fifty years of watching my children grow up and go on to have great families and careers. I have celebrated a long and wonderful life with my husband—the life I had always imagined. Moreover, I have been truly blessed with many enduring friendships that I have come to cherish with all my heart. This is my desire for you—to live every day in thankfulness, remembering not the battle but the joy of life lived to the fullest.

At the center of my "Circle of Hope" is my Lord and Savior Jesus Christ. He has been my Counselor, my Encourager, my Sustainer, and my Hope

Reflections

through this entire ordeal. I cannot imagine ever making this journey without His love and comfort, and it is my reunion with Him when the journey is over that lifts my eyes and gives me wings! Listen to these wonderful words that describe the wondrous promises He has for each of us as we finish the race: "He will wipe every tear from their eyes, and there will be no more death or sorrow or crying or pain. All these things are gone forever" (Revelation 21:4).

My friend, if you are struggling with this disease, I invite you to join with me and take up the fight to live each day to its fullest. We can and will make every day and every moment count, enjoying the unselfish love of our God, our families, and our friends. My personal prayer for you, beloved, is that He will bless you with the comfort, faith, and encouragement that I myself have received and that He will so fill your life with love that you can't help but share it with others.

In His Love,

Rena

Epilogue

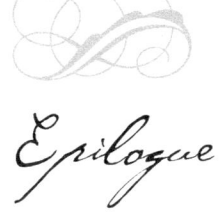

Just One More Thing

It is late afternoon on Christmas day as I write these final words to you. Bringing each page to life brought with it the unexpected gift of reliving many wonderful memories. As each memory unfolds, I see the many faces of friends and family and am overjoyed for the love that we share. These are true gifts that cause my heart and spirit to take flight, and they can never be taken away. It is a sobering thought, realizing that these are significant elements of my life that might never have been if it were not for the choices I had made those many years ago. Whenever I stop and consider this, I am profoundly aware of a word that holds a special place in my heart. It is a word that now fills my life and is one that I want you to be mindful of every day—*thankfulness*. And this time of year, I am filled with much thankfulness.

I have always loved the Christmas season. For me, it is a time of anticipation for the Spirit who embraces and unites us all. It is a celebration of hope and gratitude—a special time for thankfulness as we remember our Savior, our families, and all the blessings that make up our lives. I hope that you will join me in searching regularly for those things in our lives that are worthy of our thanks. Who are the people that have impacted your life in positive and loving ways? With what acts of kindness do you remember being blessed? How have these blessings changed your life for the better? Think about all of these things, my friend, and you, too, will be filled with a deep sense of gratitude. It is time, indeed, for each of us to remember, give thanks, and then become a wonderful blessing for others. Remember that, my friend, and remember that I'm with you.

Gratefully yours,

Rena

Recommended Reading

Ash, Mary Kay. *Mary Kay on People Management.* New York, NY: Warner Books, 1984.

——. *You Can Have It All: Lifetime Wisdom from America's Foremost Woman Entrepreneur.* Rocklin, CA: Prima Publishing. 1995.

——. *Miracles Happen: The Life and Timeless Principles of the Founder of Mary Kay, Inc.* New York: Quill, 2003.

Helmstetter, Shed. *What to Say When You Talk to Yourself: The Major New Breakthrough to Managing People, Yourself, and Success.* Scottsdale, AZ: Grindle Press, 1986.

Hill, Napoleon. *Think and Grow Rich.* Hollywood, CA: Wilshire Book Co., 1999.

Mandino, Og. *The Greatest Salesman in the World.* Hollywood, FL: Lifetime Books, 1996.

——, *The Twelfth Angel.* New York: Fawcett Columbine, 1993.

——, *The Spellbinder's Gift.* New York: Fawcett Columbine, 1995.

McNally, David. *Even Eagles Need a Push: Learning to Soar in a Changing World.* New York: Delacorte Press, 1991.

Recommended Reading

Minrith, Frank and Paul Meier, *Happiness Is a Choice: A Manual on the Symptoms, Causes, and Cures of Depression.* Grand Rapids: Baker Book House, 1978.

Newman, Mildred. *How to Be Your Own Best Friend: A Conversation with Two Psychoanalysts.* New York, Random House, 1971.

Ogilvie, Lloyd. *Making Stress Work for You: Ten Proven Principles.* Waco, TX: Word Books, 1984.

Simonton, Carl, et al., *Getting Well Again: A Step-by-Step, Self-Help Guide to Overcoming Cancer for Patients and Their Families.* Los Angeles: Jeremy Tarcher; New York: St. Martin's, 1978.

Swindoll, Charles R. *Living Above the Level of Mediocrity: A Commitment to Excellence.* Waco, TX: Word Books, 1987.

Tarbet, Rena. *Rena: How to Succeed in Spite of Life's Challenges.* Franklin, TN: Legacy Books, 1998.

Ziglar, Zig. *Over the Top.* Nashville: Thomas Nelson, 1994.

——. *Something to Smile About: Encouragement and Inspiration for Life's Ups and Downs.* Nashville: Thomas Nelson, 1997.

——. *Raising Positive Kids in a Negative World.* Nashville: Oliver Books.

About the Author

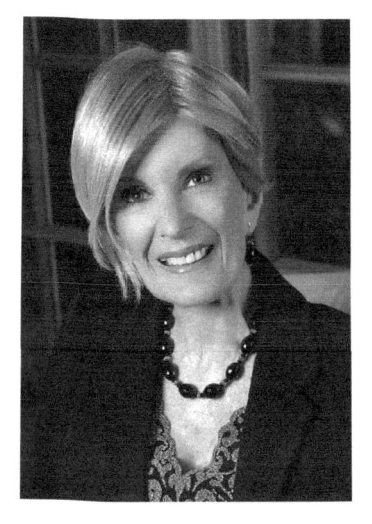

Rena Tarbet is a woman who knows what she wants and goes after it, even in the worst of circumstances. Her strength and courage are unparalleled. She lives every day with cancer and has had numerous surgeries, extensive treatments, and has endured six straight years of chemotherapy.

Even in the midst of a struggle for her life, Rena continues to work her business with the love and support of her family, which now includes three children, their spouses, and nine beautiful grandchildren.

As a Mary Kay Director, Rena surpassed all company records both in her personal sales and team production, leading the number one team in the entire company to million-dollar status four years in a row. She has now ascended to the elite position of National Sales Director Emeritus.

Rena was recognized as "Fort Worth Woman of the Year" in 1985, being featured in numerous magazines and books, including, Survivors: Living with Cancer. She is a dynamic speaker for the American Cancer Society and provides extensive counseling for cancer patients throughout the country, as well as training and empowering thousands of business professionals around the world.

In 2006, the prominent Cancer Centers Associates named their new state-of-the-art cancer center in McKinney, Texas, the Rena Tarbet Cancer Center for her lifelong dedication to cancer education and supporting and empowering patients to take control of their health and their lives to overcome the disease. Her portrait hangs in the Center's lobby, reminding every patient that they, too, can overcome cancer.

Rena is truly a legend, the epitome of strength and determination, which comes from her love for life, her family, and God. She's charming, she's daring, and she's unstoppable!